SELF-NAVIGATE FOR HEALTH

by

UCHENNA NJIAJU, MD, FACP

DISCLAIMER:

Details about medical symptoms, diagnoses, treatments, and others used in this book are fictional. Any similarity to the history of an actual person, living or dead, is purely coincidental. Please note that the medical information I share is meant to be a general guide, not a substitute for medical advice from your physician. My writing is not meant to serve as a "second or third or other opinion." My writing here is not intended to establish a physician-patient relationship. The exact approach in treating a medical condition in any particular condition depends on many variables, so please be sure to discuss your thoughts and questions with your physician. Views here are mine alone, and are not affiliated with my employer. For my medical writing here, on my blog, or on any other social media site, either under my formal name, Uchenna O. Njiaju, or under my social media name, Erica OncMD or EricaOncMD, please visit the home page of https://www.ericaoncologymd.com and read my full disclaimer.

I dedicate this book to my parents,
Prof Richard N. Okagbue and Mrs. Rose N. Okagbue.
Without their unwavering love, dedication, hard work,
and sacrifice, I would be nothing.

TABLE OF CONTENTS:

SELF-NAVIGATE ON YOUR HEALTH CARE JOURNEY

Do you have a medical illness or several? You may find it overwhelming, trying to keep up with tests, changes in medications, other doctors you are sent to see (referrals), next steps to remember. Perhaps you are lucky to have excellent health but you wonder what you should do to remain in that state. You may wish you had someone to guide and direct you. In some places, there may be professional nurse navigators who can help with this. The reality, though, is that most people do not have access to such navigators.

You may ask, "How can I help myself, or my friend or a family member? Are there any helpful tips or suggestions? How can I stay on top of things and make sure I am getting the most out of my journey? How do I make the best of each visit with my physician? How do I know what symptoms to look out for, and when to call my physician?"

I have been a physician for the past fourteen years, and I know that anyone can learn to be his or her own guide. Put simply, **anyone** can learn to *self-navigate for health*.

When I use the word "self-navigate," I mean, "take charge of your health and do all you can to prevent or delay health problems, and if they occur, make sure you get the most out of your health journey."

In this book, I share a few pointers for self-navigation and getting the most out of your medical care. After reading through the following chapters and working through the exercises, you will be convinced, confident and able to take charge of your health journey.

Here's what you'll learn:

1. That you can learn to self-navigate
2. 4 things everyone should know about their health condition
3. Why you should have a health summary

4. How to never again leave your doctors office without all questions asked and answered
5. 3 reasons to always take a notebook to a doctor appointment
6. 4 ways to know if you have a serious symptom or not
7. How to never again wonder when/whether to call your doctor
8. 4 things to think of before asking Dr. Google again
9. What to do during a medical crisis

YOU CAN LEARN TO SELF-NAVIGATE:

When you think of a navigator, you might imagine someone experienced and trustworthy, using instruments and maps, guiding a ship or aircraft safely to its destination.

How about a navigator on your medical journey? How would you like someone to direct you, making sure you are doing all you can to stay in good health; helping you remember appointments, to take your medications, and what tests to have done; checking that you are coping?

What if you can't find one? Well, you *can* learn to self-navigate!

One particular paper defines a *cancer patient navigator* (for example) as "an individual trained to help identify and resolve real and perceived barriers to care, enabling patients to adhere to care recommendations and thus improve their cancer outcomes."[1]

Whether or not you have a professional navigator, and whether or not you have any significant medical problems, it is crucial to learn how to self-navigate. If you are a caregiver for family members with complex health issues (children, parents, spouses, etc.), this is an indispensable skill.

Here are just nine steps to get you started:

1. **Sign up for health benefits:** You may be a healthy thirty-year-old who just got their first job. Perhaps you've never been sick in your whole life. That is not enough reason to overlook signing up for health insurance or that critical illness benefit offered by your employer. Money spent on safeguarding health and ensuring support if illness were to happen is money well spent. If you have dependents, make sure you sign up for as many medical, dental, and vision benefits as possible. My personal opinion is that health

benefits are important enough to forego that annual vacation or other luxury in order to have. Just like we all endeavor to have renters' insurance and life insurance, be prepared for a rainy day in regard to your health.

2. **Your primary doctor is your first and most important partner in self-navigating to health:** The Dutch philosopher Desiderius Erasmus said, "Prevention is better than cure." He lived from 1466 to 1536, and yet, several centuries later with complex and effective tools for disease diagnosis and many treatments available, his words still hold true. If I had a penny for every time I heard, "I'm always healthy and don't need doctors," I'd be a millionaire by now. In every culture, the most prominent celebrities, politicians, institutions, and businesses have a team of attorneys on staff because of the very real threat of litigation and because of other legal and regulatory issues that come up. **In the**

same light, EVERYONE is at risk of health problems, and so EVERYONE needs a doctor. Make sure you have a medical team on your side when you are healthy, and don't wait for a time of crisis. Have a primary doctor and see them at least once a year. This is something we do more for children (who need doctor's notes and immunization records for school and daycare), but adults particularly need to pay attention to this. Your primary doctor will ask about your diet and exercise habits. They will ask about your family history in order to determine what conditions you may be at risk for. They have a network of specialist doctors they can contact quickly in an emergency, on your behalf. They are connected to pharmacists, therapists, and hospitals. If you had an urgent medical issue suddenly come up, being already established with a primary doctor might mean that you get care within hours or days, rather than weeks or months when things have a chance to get much worse. Having a regular doctor means that you don't have to end up in the ER and get admitted for a problem that can be tackled in the office. Your primary doctor is focused on preventing illnesses from developing, and if they do, diagnosing them early when they are easier to treat and cure.

3. **Write, write, and write some more:** Keep a health summary. Learn and write down essentials of your medical condition(s). No, I do not mean to imply that one becomes a doctor if not trained as one, but one can come up with a short summary for reference. Keep a list of medications. Keep an account of symptoms, onset, and duration, in between appoint-ments. Keep a list of doctors and their addresses and phone numbers (and include what each doctor does; for example, Dr. X is a cardiologist who manages my heart problems). Never walk into a doctor appointment without a written agenda, and never leave without a written summary of next steps.

4. **Ask lots of questions:** Your medical team wants to know if you are uncertain about your condition or treatment plan. They are there to help you. If you forget something, do call back and ask. If you are sent to see another doctor, like an outside referral for a problem, and you don't hear back to schedule the appointment, do call. If you had a test and did not hear about results, call the office and ask. When you are told of results, ask, "What is the next step?" At appointments, do not hesitate to state if instructions are confusing, or if you need more clarification. If you get home and realize you don't understand what was discussed, call and ask for a return appointment.

5. **Disclose in full and provide updates:** Remember that so many things can cause every single symptom or test finding. Some findings can be watched, while others may need treatment now. It will help your doctor to know your prior history, your family

history, your medications, any herbs or recreational drugs you use, and some personal habits. Illnesses can run in families. A breast lump in a thirty-year-old woman may be more likely to be cancer if her mother and several maternal aunts had breast cancer. Someone who uses some recreational drugs may be more likely to have heart blood vessels constrict, causing something like a heart attack. These are a few examples. Of course such a list can be quite extensive, but most doctor's offices have forms one can fill in. It is important to be truthful and as detailed as possible.

6. **Make a habit of reporting back if not improving:** In medical school, I recall being told, "Common things are common." This means that a fifteen-year-old with shortness of breath after exercise may be treated for asthma, which is more likely than a blood clot in the lungs. On the other hand, a seventy-year-old man with the same symptom who never had it before in his life

is more likely to have a blood clot than asthma. Still, if the initial treatment does not help, it is important to report back immediately. Your doctor wants to know that you are feeling better with his/her prescribed treatment, and if not, he/she wants to know in order to consider other possibilities. It is important to remember that every single symptom can be caused by several possible conditions.

7. **Follow through and always seek closure:** If your condition is not getting better with treatment, ask your doctor what to do. If you have had several symptoms for a while and there is no diagnosis yet, ask if a second opinion might help. If a symptom happened and was unusual to you, don't ignore it just because it went away. Be sure to discuss it with your doctor. A minor headache that has happened on and off for years may not be too alarming, but a sudden episode of new slurred speech that came and went may be the beginnings of a massive

stroke. If your doctor said he/she would refer you to another doctor and you did not hear about an appointment two weeks later, call the office and ask. If you are asked to make another appointment in three months and somehow you did not make it on your way out, then plug a reminder into your calendar to call later. Do not assume that things sort themselves out.

8. **Remember other members of your health team:** If you have financial issues, a social worker can be a helpful resource. A clinical pharmacist at your doctor's office (if there is one) may be able to assist you if you are confused about medications. The scheduler is the person you contact if you need an appointment. It may be that you contact your doctor's medical assistant if you are not being called back about a referral. Put together a list of names, positions, and phone numbers for reference.

9. **Have copies of your medical records:**
This may not necessarily apply to everyone. If you have had medical tests like scans or blood tests, it is helpful to have your records with you. If you have long-term medical conditions or have had hospitalizations, this is particularly important. Your doctor's office or hospital has a medical record department where you can request records. For X-rays and scans, you should request the report, as well as the actual pictures (usually would be stored for you on a CD). You can put these away in a folder and keep it at home. If traveling for long periods of time, consider taking the folder along with you. If you are internet savvy and you have access to a patient portal where you can view your medical records, it is helpful to have an account if you have medical issues going on.

Exercise #1:

Have you signed up for health insurance? What are your options? How about revising or adding to your plan? Do you know when you can do this (usually at open enrollment twice a year in the USA)?

Exercise #2:

Who is your primary doctor? Endeavor to have his/her name, address, and phone number. Are you confident that you would know how to contact your doctor at any time of the day or night, if an issue came up? What is the number for your doctor's medical records department? Ask for your medical records and put them together in a folder to keep at home.

4 THINGS EVERYONE SHOULD KNOW ABOUT THEIR HEALTH CONDITION

Does it matter if you just go along on your health journey, doing what you're asked to do without taking time to understand some facts? The answer is a resounding yes. It does matter, and can be detrimental to your health. It is recognized that people who pay more attention and stay engaged may do better with their medical care.

Why?

The reason is because the more engaged patient has some knowledge of their health condition, asks questions, tries hard to follow recommendations, may be looking out for the most recent and applicable research, and may be challenging their medical team to consider changes in treatment if necessary, etc. While one does not have to aim at becoming a "star patient" necessarily, there are four things I have found to be important, that everyone with a chronic medical condition should know, so they can optimize their health and medical care.

1. **The name of the condition, spelling, and such basics:** Knowing more enables one to pay attention to the press, learning what's new in research and treatment. People who know more are able to better advocate for themselves in asking their doctor about treatment options, whether things need to change, etc. One may learn about experts in a particular field, potentially for a second opinion if the need ever arises. For example, someone with a rare kind of cancer may benefit from a second opinion from an expert who focuses only on that kind of cancer. Some basics one could look up include risk factors for a condition, whether inherited or not,

treatments, complications, prognoses, ongoing research, etc.

2. **When to call, and what symptoms may be worrisome:** Some symptoms like blood in stool, crushing left-sided chest pain, persistent vomiting, weakness on one side of the body, etc. are universally concerning. However, there are also symptoms that are particularly alarming for each individual, based on their medical history. For example, if you have had a prior heart attack, even a slight chest pain can be worrisome. If you have had a mastectomy for breast cancer, then a new lump on your chest wall cannot be ignored. Endeavor to discuss with your doctor and find out what symptoms are particularly worrisome in your situation.

3. **Names of medications and what each is for:** For each chronic condition, there may be a number of medications used to slow the course, treat symptoms, improve quality of life, and prevent complications.

For example, a woman undergoing chemotherapy for breast cancer may have pain medications to use if having body pains from the treatment, as well as other medications to prevent nausea. Knowing that ondansetron is for nausea means that a woman who has had lot of nausea cannot afford to run out of ondansetron. A diabetic may run out of Lipitor (used to control cholesterol to prevent stroke and heart attack) for a day or even a week, but cannot afford to run out of insulin for even a day (since serious complications can arise with high blood sugars).

4. **Any important lifestyle habits to avoid, or adopt:** By changing lifestyle habits, some conditions can be better controlled. For example, a diabetic should work on dieting and exercise for weight loss and should cut down on alcohol. A breast cancer survivor should stop postmenopausal hormone replacement therapy. Someone with hemochromatosis (a condition that

causes a buildup of iron in the body) should avoid eating raw shellfish.

HAVE A HEALTH SUMMARY

Have you ever wondered how to keep track of medical conditions, medications, etc.? Maybe for you, or a loved one, your parent or a child? Well, wonder no more. I have come up with a short and very simple guide you can use to keep things organized. I have used a hypothetical patient who has diabetes mellitus and high cholesterol just to illustrate.

The very same template below is used in the blank worksheet at the end of this book. For some people, health history may be simple enough to commit to memory.

MY HEALTH SUMMARY

My name and date of birth:

What (medical diagnoses):
Type 2 Diabetes Mellitus (DMII)
High cholesterol

More about it (no more than three phrases describing each):

Type 2 diabetes mellitus: body does not respond well to my own insulin or is resistant to it, can cause high sugar levels, predisposition to stroke, heart attack, and other organ damage in the long run

High cholesterol: too much bad cholesterol (also called LDL) can predispose to stroke, heart attack, blood vessel disease

Medications:

Name of medication	Dose	What for	How important
Lantus insulin	20 units injected under skin at night	Diabetes	Crucial
Atorvastatin	20mg by mouth at bedtime	High cholesterol	Important
Vitamin D	1000 units by mouth in the morning	To supplement vitamin D	Important
Aspirin	81 mg by mouth daily	To prevent heart attack and stroke	Important
Multivitamin	1 tablet by mouth daily	Supplement	Optional
Herbal supplement	1 tablet by mouth daily	Supplement	Optional

Allergies: Penicillin causes a rash and tongue swelling (anaphylaxis)

What I need to tell my family members:

DMII and high cholesterol can both run in families. My children may be at risk also. This shared risk can be due to genetics and/or family habits.

Important lifestyle implications:

It is important to control weight, exercise, control cholesterol and simple sugars in diet, watch salt intake. It is also important to avoid/minimize alcohol and avoid smoking, as these habits can also add to organ damage. Pay attention to feet, as ulcers can occur related to diabetic nerve and blood vessel damage. Report those immediately.

Other useful information or websites:

https://www.cdc.gov/diabetes/home/index.html
www.diabetes.org

Exercise #1:

Using the worksheet at the end of the book, write up your health summary. Plan to take a copy to your next medical appointment and check details with your doctor. Keep a copy in your medical folder.

NEVER AGAIN LEAVE YOUR DOCTOR'S OFFICE WITHOUT ALL QUESTIONS ASKED AND ANSWERED:

Even I have found myself in this situation. You anticipate your doctor appointment for weeks, have a mental list of what to ask and mention, and then you arrive and find that one particular issue (or two) takes over the visit. You get sidetracked and arrive home, only to realize that you forgot to raise another important issue. Your doctor misses out on an opportunity to address issues that might be very important for your health. For example, your doctor might ask you to take a pill to help your heartburn get better, but if he/she knows you had tarry black stools three weeks ago, he/she will likely send you immediately to have a test called *upper endoscopy.* Of course, some situations may not be as serious.

It is my opinion that everyone should have a written agenda for each doctor appointment. This is particularly important for people with complex medical issues, but I feel that everyone could benefit from such.

Chances are that when you decide to meet a realtor to discuss buying a home, you have some idea of what you want, a list on paper (ideally) or in your mind (easier to forget). When meeting that attorney for a legal issue, you also prepared in advance. In the same way, it is imperative to prepare for a doctor appointment, and here is a list one might use:

1. **Date of appointment:** This helps one remember the particular day, for reference in the future.

2. **Name and specialty of the doctor:** This is important if you see several doctors.

3. **Contact information for the doctor:** Include phone number, fax number,

address, and name and number for the doctor's nurse and front desk scheduler.

4. **How I have been:** List symptoms you have had leading up to this visit. Mention things that happened, even if they seemed inconsequential to you. Have some idea of when and for how long. Your doctor can put these together and decide which matter, which don't, which can be watched, and which need intervention.

5. **My list of medications and herbs:** Provide an update at each visit. Did you start a new medication and then stop? Your doctor needs to know those as well. Be sure to mention the reason for stopping them also.

6. **Family and social history:** Did a young family member (<45) suddenly get diagnosed with breast cancer in the interim? Did you learn that a cousin was admitted to the hospital with some medical issue? Social history has to do with substances like alcohol, tobacco, sexual habits, work, etc.

Increased alcohol consumption can explain why liver enzymes are suddenly high on a blood test.

7. **Recommendations and plan for today:** Leave some space to write down what you need to do. It could be medications to take, new lifestyle changes to try, other doctors to see, tests to have done, etc. Your doctor may give you an after-visit summary you can also file away with your paperwork. If you have tests and referrals scheduled, plug them into your calendar so as not to forget.

The more your doctor knows, the more he or she can help you. Yes, if you have a particularly lengthy agenda, your doctor might suggest tackling some items that day, and returning for another visit. Regardless, you can be sure that you will have a more productive visit that way.

Exercise #1:

Practice writing an agenda for your next medical appointment. Use the worksheet at the end of this book and take it along to your appointment.

3 REASONS TO ALWAYS TAKE A NOTEBOOK TO A DOCTOR APPOINTMENT

You have a few health issues, or more; some mild, maybe some significant. You take some medications, you have tests scheduled, and you have other issues to discuss every once in a while to stay in good health. You see your doctor every few weeks, or months. Unfortunately, you only have a few minutes. Sometimes you walk out and remember one more thing you should have asked, or you get home and realize you are confused about some issue or instruction. Sound familiar?

Believe it or not, you are not alone. I meet several like you every day. As a cancer and blood doctor, I often engage in life-altering discussions. As a mother and daughter, I have been on the other end of things, accompanying family members with significant health issues to appointments. I have figured out three reasons why taking a notebook along can help you make the most of your doctor appointment.

1. **Your written agenda will lead the discussion:** Your doctor may have some questions to ask at your appointment, but he/she really cares most about your agenda; i.e., what is troubling YOU the most? When you have notes written down, that takes the forefront and he/she can focus on those rather than a generic set of questions. Yes, you have diabetes and your doctor wants to ask whether you have noticed nerve pain in your feet or vision problems, but what if you have new-onset impotence? What if you had transient calf pain while working out a week prior? What if you are a young woman who has a new partner and may be planning a pregnancy within a year? Those are not issues your doctor is likely to guess, and you

may forget if you do not keep a running list and take it along to your appointment.

2. **You will remember details better:** This is because you will write down every confusing word, and while doing so will ask for spellings and more explanations. One could look up more details on reliable websites afterward, and can discuss better with family and friends. Writing also helps one remember instructions, and in what order. Follow-up is less likely to be missed and understanding is enhanced.

3. **The doctor-patient confidence is better:** When you write, you are more engaged during the visit. As the patient, you are more likely to walk away satisfied that your concerns were addressed. Your doctor may feel more confident that instructions and explanations were understood. Care and follow-up are better overall, particularly in complex medical situations.

SERIOUS SYMPTOM OR NOT? 4 SUGGESTIONS TO HELP

How do I know what symptom is concerning? I can't tell you how many times I have heard, "I didn't call my doctor because I didn't know it was serious." Many people Google symptoms to figure out what the cause could be. Then they try to determine what to do based on that. I've been in medicine since 1999, but even I get thoroughly confused when I look up symptoms on the internet. Every single symptom can represent dozens of problems. How then might a non-medically-trained person know what is serious and what isn't?

Well, stay with me here and you'll find out. I won't bother you with a long list of "if this, then that." I won't even list any symptoms. I have just four suggestions that will help you figure out any situation.

1. **Remember that health summary:** Having a health summary and updating it at each doctor appointment will serve as a reminder. Always ask your doctor what symptoms to look out for. A person treated for a heart attack wants to report pain in their calves with walking (could indicate disease of the blood vessels in the legs, which can present a risk of sudden blood vessel blockage that can lead to amputation if severe). Someone who has been treated for a kind of cancer called lymphoma wants to report unusual fever or night sweats. Your doctor knows your situation well and can list a few symptoms to watch out for.

2. **A few simple instructions always hold true:** No matter how small a problem might seem, if it isn't getting better, it's probably helpful to call your doctor. If a symptom persists and new problems develop, it might also indicate something more serious. For example, a minor pain in the toe can be

watched, but if the toe turns blue-black or red that can mean more. A young twenty-something-year-old woman can take Tylenol (or acetaminophen) for a headache, but if she suddenly has blurry vision, she should call. Another simple instruction is that something new and persistent needs to be looked at. If a forty-year-old suddenly has headaches (never before in the past), they should call.

3. **When in doubt, call your doctor's office:** Your doctor isn't there only for appointments. He/she has a staff (usually nurses) that can help you figure out what symptoms are worrisome and which aren't. It is always unfortunate to learn that someone waited for weeks because they had an appointment coming up, when a serious problem was actually going on. Pick up the phone, call, and ask. Your doctor's office staff will help you prioritize.

4. **Here's where Dr. Google might scare rather than help:** Remember to be careful looking up symptoms on the internet. Yes, you may get lucky and fall upon an accurate list of possible conditions. More likely though, you'll be overwhelmed and confused. Dr. Google is more helpful for general information, rather than specific advice for a situation.

Exercise #1:

Do you have a list of symptoms to look out for in your unique situation? If not, ask your doctor at your next appointment. If you do not have an appointment coming up soon, consider calling your doctor's office to ask. Write the list down in your health summary.

NEVER AGAIN WONDER WHEN/WHETHER TO CALL YOUR DOCTOR:

Let's face a fact. You get to see your doctor for fifteen minutes or so every couple of weeks or months. Maybe you see him/her once a year. That is not a lot of time. It may not matter if you don't have much going on health-wise. What if you have several health issues though or you're taking several medications? What if you have complications that come up occasionally? Do you wonder how to stay connected with your doctor without feeling like a bother? Do you wonder when it is appropriate to call and when to wait?

Here are four things to keep in mind:

1. **It really is okay to call if you need to.** Most of the time, you might need to call in between appointments if you have a serious question. For example, you may be out of your medications or having a side effect from a new medication. Perhaps you have a new symptom. Maybe you remembered that you need to have a foot exam once a year and called to check. Maybe you feel you should be getting a mammogram before your next appointment and decided to call and ask. In other words, a question or concern that you need to clarify before your next appointment is a good enough reason to call. The best health care involves an attentive doctor and an engaged patient.

2. **It does help if you try to prioritize.** If you realize on a Friday afternoon that your medication runs out in a week, it is okay to wait and call on Monday, unless it takes a long time to get a new supply. If you notice that your toenail is turning a bit brown and

there is no pain or bleeding or fever, you could wait for your scheduled appointment the following week. The same applies to new heartburn. On the other hand, sudden onset headache in a sixty-year-old who has never had headaches is a good reason to call immediately, even at 8:00 p.m. Of course, a non-medically-trained person might be uncertain of a few things. That is where the expertise of your doctor and his/her staff comes in handy. One should try to prioritize, but whenever uncertain, it is best to err on the side of caution. Your doctor's office staff (usually nurses) can tell you when to come in immediately, and when to wait a few days or even weeks.

3. **Staying in touch is good for your health.** Once in a while, health problems are dramatic, but mostly they start slowly and then get worse over time. This means that calling your doctor early allows him or her to intervene before things get out of

hand. If you are on chemotherapy, for example, it is more useful to call immediately if nausea is not responding to medications. Your oncologist may schedule intravenous fluids and intravenous medications that can help pretty quickly. After two to three days of nausea and vomiting all day, one might have dehydration and malfunctioning kidneys and may need hospital admission. In fact, a recent study confirmed that cancer patients who self-report symptoms do better and live longer.[2]

4. **Other updates are equally important.** What if you are traveling and need medical care? What if you end up in an emergency room or urgent care center on a weekend? Your doctor really does need to know. Your health complication may matter for your future care. As soon as you are able to, it is important to call your doctor's office and notify them of the event. It is helpful to have

the name of the hospital and dates so that your doctor can request records. It is also important to take note of any new medications that were prescribed, and to remember whatever was diagnosed if possible. Usually, an emergency room doctor provides a summary note that can help.

BEFORE ASKING DR. GOOGLE AGAIN, THINK OF THESE FOUR THINGS:

Have you been on Google lately? Maybe for health reasons you like to check causes of chest pain, diarrhea, and fainting; examples of treatments for a sore throat; side effects of medications? The list is endless. If you are like most people I encounter, you may feel quite armed with the medical information on the internet. You may feel like you have an idea about most things, you know what can cause some symptoms, and some things to do for a number of health problems. Right?

Wrong.

Let me start by saying that each human being, every situation, and every point in time are all unique. Diabetes can look a hundred different ways and be managed a hundred different ways. Breast cancer is a hundred different diseases. If you read the side effect profile of Tylenol and learn that people die from an overdose of this medication every year, you might hesitate before you open your medicine cabinet to take a tablet (or two) for a headache tonight.

This is why everyone should approach his or her doctor for a bothersome health concern. Dr. Google IS NOT, and SHOULD NEVER be a substitute for medical care by a trained and licensed physician.

Still, sometimes one may need to look something up, to understand better or to get more information. The internet really is a good thing and can be helpful at such times, as long as one pays attention to three points:

1. **Be careful with non-medical authors and chat forums.** How many times have you received service from a hotel, or store, or restaurant, and received yet another survey? How many have you completed and sent back? I bet you that you've completed

more where you had something really great (or really bad) to say, right? This is why I always advise caution with blogs and other forums where the non-medical public discusses health issues. Consider that you may not be hearing from the larger average population, but rather you might be focusing on the experience of the outliers. Also, if you want information about chicken breeding, I suspect you would want to check poultry farm websites rather than a website with chicken entree recipes. The expertise does matter.

2. **Know the dependable sites.** It makes sense to verify the background of the author whenever you are reading medical information on the internet. Because of their sheer size and reputation, you can be sure that information posted by large health institutions is reliable and accurate. Some examples include the Mayo Clinic and National Institutes of Health. University

(.edu) and government (.gov) websites are also reliable.

3. **Remember that geography does matter.** A streptococcal (strep) sore throat is the same no matter where you go, but antibiotics may be named differently. In some complex areas like cancer care, the treatment approach can vary quite a bit from place to place. It makes sense to seek out reputable authors practicing in your particular part of the world first, before looking elsewhere.

4. **General information is more useful.** Because every person and situation is different, it is unwise to expect that every complication listed may apply to you, or that your case will go a certain way exactly. It is more beneficial to read about the different types of breast cancer, like ER/PR positive and HER2 positive, rather than expecting that you will get TCH chemotherapy

necessarily just because you have HER2-positive breast cancer and someone else on a chat forum got the same.

Exercise #1:

Do you know what websites have the most dependable information for your medical situation? Does your doctor's office have information posted online, perhaps on a blog? Endeavor to find out and keep such a list of websites handy.

WHAT TO DO DURING A MEDICAL CRISIS OR IF THERE IS A COMPLICATION:

Alas, most of us have to face this at one time or another. It may be personal, or a friend or family member. One who was completely healthy may suddenly fall ill, or a longstanding medical condition may get worse. There may be warning signs or not; worsening may be unexpected or not. We may find ourselves supporting an adult, an elderly loved one, or a child. Hospital admission may even be required. As challenging as such times can be, you can self-navigate for health during a medical crisis by following just nine steps outlined below. Loved ones can be very helpful with these since the sick person may be too unwell to help him or herself.

1. **Trust your instincts.** Guess what? No one knows your body better than you, not even your doctor with years or decades of medical training and work experience. You know how you feel most of the time, and so you know best when something is wrong. Your doctor may see you for a rash and diagnose an allergic reaction, but what if two days later you feel weaker and have a poor appetite? Be sure to call your doctor and discuss the new symptoms you are feeling. It might make a difference between continuing to watch you at home versus getting some blood tests to see if something serious is going on. As a parent, I would add that the same applies to young children under our care. If you feel something is not right, you are probably correct. Call that pediatrician back and insist they check the child again. If you are not satisfied with their response, look for another doctor perhaps at another pediatrician office, or urgent care, or emergency room. Do not hesitate to go back ten times if you are not satisfied. It is better

to end up being wrong than to miss something serious.

2. **Call your doctor early and get some guidance.** Certainly, we all have symptoms come up once in a while that we watch for a bit. What I mean here is that once you feel something is unusual, get in touch with your doctor. If you have a minor cold, you can take something over the counter and watch for it to get better. If it doesn't get better and you start coughing up blood on a Friday, don't wait for Monday to call. Remember that your doctor's office has someone covering over the weekend. Call them and ask what to do. Use your doctor's expertise to help you prioritize, rather than trying to guess or looking on Google.

3. **Keep a timeline.** Doctors are human too. In a complex and protracted medical situation, you may have many doctors get involved at different times. After a while, it

may become increasingly difficult to remember what happened when. We all get stressed in a medical crisis and may forget details. Nowadays, many of us have smartphones and email. Here's where electronics can come in handy. In a medical crisis, it helps to write what happens day to day. Did the fever start before the rash? Did you notice blood in the stool on the first or third day? Write short paragraphs per day. Write what happened, which doctor you saw, what they said, what tests were done, what treatments were given. Write in short sentences and enter a date for each day. Some treatments cause side effects, and timelines can help your doctor figure out what complication is related to the illness versus due to medications or such. When new doctors get involved down the line, you can refer to the timeline to help them better understand what happened. Sometimes it takes several doctors to review a case before someone figures out a diagnosis. Keep in mind that many different people might get involved along the way and may still ask you to look back to when everything started.

4. **Take many pictures.** This can be very helpful. If you notice a new skin finding or change in color of the eyes or urine or stool, take a picture. Such a little detail can help your doctor make a diagnosis. Store pictures on your cell phone and have them available to show your doctor(s).

5. **Keep a list of medical staff you encounter:** For each doctor you encounter, ask for a name, specialty, and a contact phone number. Find a way to remember each person. It may be that you write down the date you saw them, or something they said.

6. **Ask for a second opinion:** If symptoms are not getting better, or the medical team remains uncertain of the diagnosis or how to

treat, consider asking for a second opinion. Depending on the situation, it might involve having another doctor get involved. If there is a hospitalization, remember that there may be hospitals that can provide a higher level of care in terms of more sophisticated tools for diagnosis and treatment. In most cases, these are University-based teaching hospitals where doctors are more highly sub-specialized and also perform research. One can politely request a transfer to another hospital for a loved one who is not responding to treatments.

7. **Contact your employer and remember your benefits:** This may apply to employed persons. It may help to contact the employer early, in order to notify of illness. Even a quick text or email may help. Considering that illness can get worse before it improves, the sooner this is done, the better.

8. **Decide on your support system and find a way to keep them updated:** I have already mentioned that loved ones are indispensable in times of crisis. Do you live alone and find yourself heading to the emergency room for a problem? Have you been feeling poorly and thinking you ought to see a doctor? Consider sending a text to a loved one to make sure that someone knows. Sometimes, a medical condition can suddenly worsen and someone may become incapacitated in a matter of hours or days. It helps to make sure that people who need to know are informed, so that one can have the support they need.

9. **Remember there is a recovery phase, so stay on track with the treatment plan:** Perhaps you or a loved one were admitted to hospital and then discharged. Do not assume that discharge means everything is perfectly normal. It typically means that there is no more need to keep

treating in the hospital, but treatments and follow-up need to continue in the office. There may be blood results that are still abnormal and need follow-up. There may be more tests to be done. It is important to follow up to the fullest so that the medical complication does not recur. Continue to keep a list of things that need follow-up, and ask your doctor if you are not sure of something.

WORKSHEETS:

A. MY HEALTH SUMMARY

My name and date of birth

What (medical diagnoses):

1.

2.

More about it (no more than three phrases describing each):

1.

2.

Medications:

Name	Dose	What for	How important

Allergies:

What I need to tell my family members:

1.

2.

Important lifestyle implications:

1.

2.

Other useful information or websites:

1.

2.

B. DOCTOR VISIT TEMPLATE:

Date of appointment: Month, day, and year of visit

Name of doctor and specialty: This is particularly important if you see many doctors.

Contact information for the doctor: Include phone number, fax number, address, and name and number for the doctor's nurse and front desk scheduler.

How I have been: List all symptoms you have had leading up to this visit. Include when they started or for how long they have been going on.

My list of medications and herbs: Include all prescription and over-the-counter medications, and herbs.

Family and social history: Indicate if there are any new illnesses you have learned about among your family members. Remember to mention if you have a new habit like smoking or alcohol or excess caffeine intake.

Recommendations and plan for today: Ask your doctor to summarize what you need to do after the appointment. It could be a test, or blood draw, or having to see another doctor (referral). Also indicate when you need to come back for your next appointment.

C: MEDICAL CRISIS OR COMPLICATION TIMELINE:

Date	Tests done	Doctors seen	What was said
January 1, 2018	CAT scan of belly	Doctor X, a gastroenterologist	Doctor X said _____ and suggested repeat blood tests tomorrow

ACKNOWLEDGMENTS:

I thank the Almighty God for strengthening me always with His love and grace. My gratitude goes to my husband, Ike, who is my rock, as well as my young children, who inspire me every day with their innocent enthusiasm for life. I am indebted to several individuals who encouraged me to write this book, assisted tirelessly with proofreading and editing, offered their precious time to discuss the content, and coached me through the publication steps. In particular, I'd like to thank Drs. Adeshola Ezeokoli, Anna Melissa Murillo, and Frank Ndayahoze. My fabulous author friend, Mary Zalmanek, took great pains to go over my initial manuscript in detail, and provided me with very useful information and guidance.

Over the years, numerous patients have entrusted me with their care. Every day they make me determined to do better, and I am thankful. I am grateful for my siblings and their spouses, who have all encouraged me on my writing and blogging journey, in many different ways. I am indebted to other innumerable relatives, friends, and followers on social media, whose questions always push me to rethink, to make each piece even better than the previous.

REFERENCES:

1. Braun K. L., et al. "Cancer Patient Navigator Tasks across the Cancer Care Continuum." *J Health Care Poor Underserved.* 2012 Feb 1; 23(1):398-413.

2. Basch E. M., et al. "Overall Survival Results of a Randomized Trial Assessing Patient-Reported Outcomes for Symptom Monitoring During Routine Cancer Treatment." *Proceedings from the American Society of Clinical Oncology*; June 2 – 6, 2017; Chicago, IL. Plenary Session.